HEAL YOUR ULCERS

Gastric Ulcers, Stress Ulcer, Ulcer Pain, Ulcers Relief, Food for Ulcers

(Including Ulcerative Colitis)

Him Rudram Saikia

© Rudram Publication, 2017 All rights reserved. This work may well not be translated or copied entirely or partly without the written permission of the publisher (Rudram Publication), except for brief excerpts in connection with reviews or scholarly analysis. Use in connection with any form of information storage and recovery, electronic edition, computer software, or by like or dissimilar tactic now known or hereafter developed is outlawed. The use in this publication of trade names, trademarks, service marks, and similar terms, even if they are not identified as such, is not to be taken as an expression of opinion as to whether or not they are subject to proprietary rights.

First Published: 2017

© 2017: Rudram Publication
ISBN: 9781521258545

DEDICATION

To my parents and other family members

BENEFIT AND PLAN OF THE BOOK:

Now a day, there is a common health problem among the people: that is Ulcers (commonly Stomach Ulcers). Now question is what is Ulcers? The strain of modern life or a reliable diet of junk food causes ulcers in the stomach and small intestine, however they are nonetheless common inside our society: About one from every 10 peoples are affected from the burning, gnawing stomach pain of the peptic (or gastric) ulcer sooner or later in life.

This book **Heal Your Ulcers** covers all the issues associated with Ulcers. People ask questions such as what are Ulcers, how to get rid of a Ulcers, what are the Ulcers causes, peptic or gastric ulcer, Ulcerative Colitis, relief measures, how to treat? What is Ulcers diet? This book tries to incorporate all these issues along with Ulcers free cooking and natural ways of treating Ulcers. It is not a book of medication of Ulcers and all those suggestions are collected from patients facing Ulcers. We hope that all these will help to cure Ulcers or to prevent Ulcers. So do not miss the opportunity to cure Ulcers. We ensure that this book will help you to know 80% of the issues related to Ulcers.

CONTENTS

Chapter - 1
Introduction to Ulcers

Chapter - 2
Peptic Ulcers

Chapter - 3
Identify the Symptoms of Belly Ulcers

Chapter -4
Changing Your Daily Diet

Chapter - 5
Making Changes in Lifestyle

Chapter - 6
Treat Ulcers Naturally

Chapter - 7
Steps To Make Cabbage Juice

Chapter - 8
Staying Away From Few Foods

Chapter - 9
Home Cures for a Belly Ulcer

Chapter – 10
Ulcerative Colitis

CHAPTER - 1

INTRODUCTION TO ULCERS

There is absolutely no clear evidence to claim that the strain of modern life or a reliable diet of junk food causes ulcers in the stomach and small intestine, however they are nonetheless common inside our society: About one from every 10 peoples are affected from the burning, gnawing stomach pain of the peptic (or gastric) ulcer sooner or later in life. Peptic ulcers are cracks or fractures in the shielding lining of the duodenum or the belly - areas with connection to abdomen acids & enzymes. Duodenal ulcers are more prevalent than belly ulcers. Comparatively uncommon are esophageal ulcers, which form in the esophagus or swallowing tube and tend to be due to contact with medications, like certain anti-inflammatories or antibiotics, or alcoholic beverages abuse.

Before 1980s, the conformist insight was that ulcers form accordingly of tension, a inherited tendency to extreme gastric acid emission, & poor routine practice (including overindulge in well-off and oily foods, alcohol, caffeine, and tobacco). It had been thought that such affects donate to an accumulation of abdomen acids that rot the protective lining of the tummy, duodenum, or esophagus.

While excessive gastric acid emission surely is significant in the opening of ulcers, a recent theory finds that infectivity is the origin cause of peptic ulcers. Indeed, research conducted because the mid-1980s shows that the bacterium Helicobacter pylori(H. pylori) exists in more than 90% of duodenal ulcers and about

80% of belly ulcers. However, newer numbers indicate those percentages are declining.

Other factors also appear to contribute to ulcer formation. Overuse of over-the-counter painkillers (such as aspirin, ibuprofen, and naproxen), heavy alcoholic beverages use, mental stress, and smoking exacerbate and could promote the introduction of ulcers, in someone with H especially pylori.

Other studies also show that abdomen ulcers will develop in the elderly. This can be because arthritis is common in older people, and alleviating arthritis pain often means taking daily doses of aspirin or ibuprofen. Another adding factor may be that with improving age group the pylorus (the valve between your tummy and duodoneum) relaxes and allows extra bile (a substance stated in the liver organ to assist in digestive function) to seep up in to the belly and rot the abdomen lining.

Also, for no known reason, people who have type A blood will develop cancerous tummy ulcers. Duodenal ulcers have a predisposition to come into view in group who have type O blood, perhaps because they don't fabricate the material on the acme of blood cells that may guard the lining of the duodenum.

Fortunately, peptic ulcers are not too difficult to treat; oftentimes they are healed with antibiotics, antacids, and other drugs that decrease the amount of acidity made by the belly. There are also a number of self-help and option treatments that can certainly help in relieving pain. Still, the risks associated with peptic ulcers such as anemia, profuse bleeding, and abdomen malignancy are serious, so ulcers should be supervised by your physician.

CHAPTER - 2

PEPTIC ULCERS

Ulcers are sores or lesions in your tummy or the top part of your small intestines. Ulcers develop when the acids that break down foods harm the belly or intestinal wall space. Connected to a number of causes like stress, diet, and lifestyle, scientists now know that lots of ulcers are the effect of a kind of bacteria called Helicobacter pylori, or H. pylori. Remaining untreated, most ulcers will continue steadily to get worse, so it is important to get an authentic diagnosis and make the diet and changes in lifestyle that will help you to heal fully.

What Exactly Are Peptic Ulcers?

1. Peptic ulcers are sores that develop in the liner of the abdomen, lower esophagus, or small intestine.

2. The most frequent sign of a peptic ulcer is burning up stomach pain that extends from the navel to the upper body.

3. Untreated ulcers may become worse as time passes and business lead to other health issues.

Peptic ulcers are sores that develop in the liner of the stomach, lower esophagus, or small intestine (the duodenum), usually because of this of inflammation caused by the bacteria H. pylori, as well as from erosion from tummy acids. Peptic ulcers are a reasonably common medical condition.

You will find three types of peptic ulcers:

- Gastric ulcers: ulcers that develop inside the stomach

- Esophageal ulcers: ulcers that develop inside the esophagus

- Duodenal ulcers: ulcers that develop in top of the section of the tiny intestines, called the duodenum

Factors behind Peptic Ulcers

Different facets can cause the liner of the belly, the esophagus, and the tiny intestine to breakdown. Included in these are:

- Helicobacter pylori (H. pylori): A bacteria that can result in a stomach contamination and inflammation

- Regular use of aspirin, ibuprofen, and other anti-inflammatory drugs (risk associated with this behavior raises in women and persons older than 60)

- Smoking

- Taking in too much alcohol

- Rays therapy

- Abdomen cancer

Symptoms of Peptic Ulcers

The most frequent symptom of a peptic ulcer is burning stomach pain that extends from the navel to the chest, which can range between mild to severe. In some full cases, the pain may wake you up during the night. Small peptic ulcers might not produce any symptoms in the early phases.

Other common signals of a peptic ulcer include:

- Changes in appetite
- Nausea
- Bloody or dark stools (melena)
- Unexplained weight loss
- Indigestion
- vomiting
- Upper body pain

Assessments and Examinations For Peptic Ulcers

Your doctor use information from your health background, a physical exam, and assessments to diagnose an ulcer and its own cause. The existence of the ulcer can only just be dependent on looking straight at the tummy with endoscopy or an X-ray test.

Medical History

To greatly help diagnose a peptic ulcer, your physician will ask you questions about your health background, your symptoms, and the medicines you take.

Make sure to point out medicines that you take without a prescription, especially non-steroidal anti-inflammatory drugs (NSAIDs), such as

- Aspirin (Bayer Aspirin)

- Ibuprofen (Motrin, Advil)

- Naproxen (Aleve)

Physical Exam

A physical exam can help a health care provider diagnose a peptic ulcer. Throughout a physical exam, a health care provider most often

- Inspections for bloating in your abdomen

- Listens to noises within your stomach utilizing a stethoscope

- Taps on your belly looking at for tenderness or pain

Lab tests

To find out if you have a Helicobacter pylori (H. pylori) illness, your physician will order these checks:

Bloodstream test:

A bloodstream test involves sketching an example of your bloodstream at the doctor's office or a commercial service. A healthcare professional testing the blood test to find out if the results fall within the standard range for different disorders or attacks.

Urea Breathing Test:

For any urea breathing test, you will drink particular water which has urea, a waste materials product that the body makes as it reduces protein. If H. pylori can be found, the bacteria changes this waste materials product into carbon dioxide-a safe gas. Skin tightening and normally shows up in your breathing when you exhale.

A healthcare professional will need an example of your breathing with you breathe into a handbag at the doctor's office or at a laboratory. She or he then sends your breathing test to a laboratory for screening. If you're breathing test has higher degrees of skin tightening and than normal, you have H. pylori in your belly or small intestine.

Stool test:

Doctors use excrement test to review an example of your stool. A health care provider will provide you with a box for catching and storing your stool at home. You come back the test to the physician or a commercial service who then sends it to a laboratory for evaluation. Stool exams can show the existence of H. pylori.

Top gastrointestinal (GI) endoscopy and biopsy

Within an upper GI endoscopy, a gastroenterologist, surgeon, or other trained healthcare professional uses an endoscope to see within your upper GI tract. This process occurs at a medical center or outpatient middle.

An intravenous (IV) needle will be positioned in your arm to give a sedative. Sedatives help you stay calm and comfortable through the process. In some instances, the procedure can be carried out without sedation. You'll be given a liquid anesthetic to gargle or aerosol anesthetic on the trunk of your throat. The physician will carefully give food to the endoscope down your esophagus and into the abdomen and duodenum. A little camera installed on the endoscope sends a video image to a monitor, allowing close study of the liner of your top GI tract. The endoscope pumps air into the tummy and duodenum, making them simpler to see.

The physician may execute a biopsy with the endoscope by firmly taking a small little bit of tissue from the liner of your esophagus. You won't feel the biopsy. A pathologist examines the cells in a laboratory.

Top GI series

An higher GI series talks about the form of your top GI tract. An x-ray specialist performs this test at a medical center or an outpatient middle. A radiologist reads and reviews on the x-ray images. You don't need anesthesia. A healthcare professional will let you know how to get ready for the task, including when to avoid eating and consuming.

Through the procedure, you'll stand or sit down before an x-ray machine and drink barium, a chalky liquid. Barium jackets your esophagus, belly, and small intestine which mean that your doctor can easily see the designs of the organs more obviously on x-rays.

You might have bloating and nausea for a short while following the test. For several times afterward, you might have white or light-colored stools from the barium. A healthcare professional will provide you with instructions about eating and consuming following the test.

Computerized Tomography (CT) scan

A CT scan uses a mixture of x-rays and computer technology to create images. For any CT scan, a healthcare professional can provide you a remedy to drink and an injection of a particular dye, which doctors call comparison medium. You'll lie on a desk that slides into a tunnel-shaped device that requires the x-rays. An x-ray specialist performs the task within outpatient middle or a medical center, and a radiologist interprets the images. You don't need anesthesia.

CT scans can help diagnose a peptic ulcer that has generated an opening in the wall structure of your abdomen or small intestine.

How exactly to treat a Peptic Ulcer

Treatment depends on the underlying reason behind your ulcer. If lab tests show you have an H. pylori infection, your doctor will prescribe a mixture of medication, which you must take for two weeks. The medications include antibiotics to help kill attacks, and proton pump inhibitors (PPIs) in reducing stomach acid.

You might experience small side results like diarrhea or upset tummy from antibiotic regimens. If these part results cause significant pain or don't progress over time, speak to your doctor.

If your physician determines that you don't have an H. pylori disease, they could recommend a prescription or over-the-counter PPI (such as Prilosec or Prevacid) for eight weeks to lessen gastric acid and help your ulcer heal.

Acid solution blockers (like Zantac or Pepcid) can also reduce gastric acid and ulcer pain. These medications can be found as a prescription and also over-the-counter in lower doses.

Complications of the Peptic Ulcer

Untreated ulcers may become worse as time passes and lead to other, much more serious health complications, such as:

• **Perforation:** A opening develops in the liner of the belly or small intestine and causes contamination. A sign of the perforated ulcer is sudden, severe stomach pain.

• **Internal bleeding:** Bleeding ulcers can lead to significant loss of blood and therefore require hospitalization. Indicators of a bleeding ulcer include lightheadedness, dizziness, and dark stools.

• **Scar tissues:** That is solid cells that evolve after a personal injury. This tissue helps it be problematic for food to feed your digestive system. Signs of scar tissue formation include vomiting and weight reduction.

All three problems are medical emergencies that want surgery. Call your physician in the event that you feel dizzy or if symptoms come back. Seek urgent medical assistance if you have the next symptoms:

• Sudden, sharp stomach pain

• Fainting, sweating, or confusion, as these may be indicators of shock

• Bloodstream in vomit or stool

• Abdominal that's hard to touch

Perspective for Peptic Ulcers

With medicine, most peptic ulcers heal. However, you might not heal if you stop taking your medication early or continue steadily to use tobacco and pain relievers during treatment. Your physicians will routine a follow-up visit after your preliminary treatment to judge your recovery.

Some ulcers, called refractory ulcers, don't heal with treatment. In case your ulcer doesn't heal with the original treatment, this may indicate:

- An excessive creation of gastric acid.

- Existence of bacteria apart from H. pylori in the stomach.

- Another disease, such as abdomen tumor or Crohn's disease.

Your physician may provide a different approach to treatment or run additional assessments to eliminate stomach cancers and other gastrointestinal diseases.

Preventing Peptic Ulcers

Certain lifestyle options and practices can lessen your threat of developing peptic ulcers. Included in these are:

- Not taking in more than two alcohol consumption a day

- Not mixing alcoholic beverages with medication

- Washing the hands frequently to avoid infections

- Restricting your use of ibuprofen, aspirin, and naproxen sodium

Maintaining a wholesome lifestyle through a well balanced diet abundant with fruits, vegetables, and wholegrain, and giving up smoking and other tobacco use will also help you prevent creating a peptic ulcer.

Just how do NSAIDs (Non-Steroidal Anti-Inflammatory Drugs) result in a peptic ulcer?

To comprehend how NSAIDs cause peptic ulcer disease, it's important to comprehend how NSAIDs work. Non-steroidal anti-inflammatory drugs decrease pain, fever, and swelling, or swelling.

Everyone has two enzymes that produce chemicals in your body's cells that promote pain, irritation, and fever. NSAIDs work by blocking or reducing the quantity of these enzymes that the body makes. However, one of the enzymes also produces a different type of chemical substance that protects the tummy lining from gastric acid and helps control bleeding. When NSAIDs stop or decrease the amount of the enzyme within you, they also boost your chance of creating a peptic ulcer.

Just how do H. pylori result in a peptic ulcer and peptic ulcer disease?

H. pylori are spiral-shaped bacteria that can cause peptic ulcer disease by damaging the mucous coating that protects the liner of the belly and duodenum. Once H. pylori have broken the mucous coating, powerful gastric acid can complete to the delicate lining. Together, the gastric acid and H. pylori irritate the liner of the abdomen or duodenum and result in a peptic ulcer.

Just how do tumors from ZES cause peptic ulcers?

Zollinger-Ellison syndrome is an uncommon disorder that occurs when a number of tumors form in your pancreas and duodenum. The tumors release huge amounts of gastric, a hormone that triggers your stomach to create huge amounts of acidity. The extra acidity causes peptic ulcers to create in your duodenum and in the top intestine.

Treatment for Peptic Ulcers (Belly Ulcers)

There are many types of medicines used to take care of a peptic ulcer. Your physician will determine the best treatment predicated on the reason for your peptic ulcer.

Just how do doctors treat an NSAID-induced peptic ulcer?

If NSAIDs are leading to your peptic ulcer and you don't have an H. pylori infection, your physician may tell you firmly to

· Stop taking the NSAID

· Reduce how a lot of the NSAID you take

· Switch to some other medication that won't result in a peptic ulcer

Your doctor could also prescribe medicines to lessen gastric acid and coating and protect your peptic ulcer. Proton pump inhibitors (PPIs), histamine receptor blockers, and protectants can help decrease pain and help your ulcer heal.

Proton pump inhibitors (PPIs)

PPIs reduce gastric acid and protect the liner of your tummy and duodenum. While PPIs can't kill H. pylori, they are doing help battle the H. pylori contamination.

PPIs include

· Esomeprazole (Nexium)

· Dexlansoprazole (Dexilant)

· Lansoprazole (Prevacid)

· Omeprazole (Prilosec, Zegerid)

· Pantoprazole (Protonix)

· Rabeprazole (Aciphex)

Histamine receptor blockers

Histamine receptor blockers work by blocking histamine, a chemical substance within you that indicators your stomach to create acid solution. Histamine receptor blockers include

- cimetidine (Tagamet)
- famotidine (Pepcid)
- ranitidine (Zantac)
- nizatidine (Axid) Protectants

Protectants

Protectants layer ulcers and protect them against acidity and enzymes so that recovery may appear. Doctors only prescribe one protectant-sucralfate (Carafate) for peptic ulcer disease.

Inform your physician if the drugs cause you to feel sick and tired or dizzy or cause diarrhea or headaches. Your doctor can transform your medicines. In the event that you smoke, quit. Additionally you should avoid alcoholic beverages. Alcohol consumption and smoking sluggish the curing of the peptic ulcer and makes it worse.

Imagine if I still need to take NSAIDs?

Invest the NSAIDs for other conditions, such as arthritis, you should talk with your doctor about the risks and benefits of using NSAIDs. Your doctor will help you determine how to keep using an NSAID securely after your peptic ulcer symptoms disappear completely. Your physician may prescribe a medication used to avoid NSAID-induced ulcers called Misoprosotol .

Tell your physician about all the prescription and over-the-counter drugs you take. Your physician can then determine if you might properly take NSAIDs or should you switch to another medicine. In either full case, your physician may prescribe a PPI or histamine receptor blocker to safeguard the liner of your belly and duodenum.

If you want NSAIDs, you can decrease the potential for a peptic ulcer returning by

· Taking the NSAID with meals

· Using the cheapest effective dosage possible

· Giving up smoking

· Staying away from alcohol

Just how do doctors treat an NSAID-induced peptic ulcer when you yourself have an H. pylori infection?

When you have an H. pylori infection, a health care provider will treat your NSAID-induced peptic ulcer with PPIs or histamine receptor blockers and other medications, such as antibiotics, bismuth subsalicylates, or antacids. PPIs reduce gastric acid and protect the liner of your abdomen and duodenum. While PPIs can't kill H. pylori, they actually help combat the H. pylori illness.

Antibiotics

A health care provider will prescribe antibiotics to kill H. pylori. How doctors prescribe antibiotics varies across the world. Over time, some types of antibiotics can't eliminate certain types of H. pylori.

Antibiotics could cure most peptic ulcers caused by H. H or pylori. Pylori-induced peptic ulcers. However, eliminating the bacteria can be difficult. Take all doses of your antibiotics just as your physician prescribes, even if the pain from a peptic ulcer is fully gone.

Bismuth subsalicylates

Medications containing bismuth subsalicylate, such as Pepto-Bismol, coating a peptic ulcer and protect it from gastric acid.

Although bismuth subsalicylate can destroy H. pylori, doctors prescribe it with antibiotics sometimes, not instead of antibiotics.

Triple therapy

For triple therapy, your physician will prescribe that you take the next for 7 to 2 weeks:

- The antibiotic clarithromycin
- The antibiotic metronidazole or the antibiotic amoxicillin
- A PPI

Quadruple therapy

For quadruple therapy, your physician will prescribe that you take the next for two weeks:

- A PPI
- Bismuth subsalicylate
- The antibiotics tetracycline and metronidazole

Doctors prescribe quadruple therapy to take care of patients who

- Can't take amoxicillin because of the allergy to penicillin. Amoxicillin and Penicillin are similar.
- Have previously received a macrolide antibiotic, such as clarithromycin.
- Are still contaminated with H. pylori after triple therapy treatment.

Doctors prescribe quadruple therapy following the first treatment has failed. In the next circular of treatment, the doctor may prescribe different antibiotics than those that he or she recommended the first time.

Sequential therapy

For sequential therapy, your physician will prescribe that you take the next for 5 times:

· A PPI

· Amoxicillin

Then your doctor will prescribe you the next for another 5 times:

· A PPI

· Clarithromycin

· The antibiotic tinidazole

Triple, quadruple, and sequential therapy could grounds sickness and other part consequences.

· An modified sense of taste

· Darkened Stools

· A darkened tongue

· Diarrhea

· Headaches

· Short-term reddening of your skin when alcohol consumption

· Vaginal yeast-based infections

Chat with your physician about any aspect results that frustrate you. She or he may prescribe you other medications.

Just how do doctors treat peptic ulcers caused by ZES?

Doctors use medications, surgery, and chemotherapy to take care of Zollinger-Ellison syndrome. Find out about Zollinger-Ellison symptoms treatment.

Imagine if a peptic ulcer doesn't heal?

Most often, medications heal a peptic ulcer. If an H. pylori disease triggered your peptic ulcer, you should end all your antibiotics and take some other medicines your physician prescribes. Chlamydia and peptic ulcer will heal only when you take all medications as your physician prescribes.

When you yourself have finished your medications, your doctor can do another breathing or stool test in four weeks or even more to make sure the H. pylori contamination is fully gone. Sometimes, H. pylori bacteria remain present, even after you have correctly taken all the medicines. If chlamydia continues to be present, your peptic ulcer could come back or, rarely, tummy malignancy could develop. Your doctor will prescribe different antibiotics to eliminate the infection and cure your peptic ulcer.

Can a peptic ulcer keep coming back?

Yes, a peptic ulcer will come back. In the event that you smoke or take NSAIDs, peptic ulcers will come back. If you want to take an NSAID, your physician may change you to a new medication or add medications to assist in preventing a peptic ulcer. Peptic ulcer disease can come back, even though you have been careful to lessen your risk.

How do I prevent a peptic ulcer?

To greatly help prevent a peptic ulcer triggered by NSAIDs, ask your physician should you

· Stop using NSAIDS

· Take NSAIDS with meals if you nevertheless still need nsaids

· Take a lesser dosage of NSAIDS

· Take medicines to safeguard your belly and duodenum while taking NSAIDS

· Change to a medication that won't cause ulcers

To greatly help prevent a peptic ulcer triggered by H. pylori, your physician may advise that you avoid alcohol consumption.

CHAPTER - 3

IDENTIFY THE SYMPTOMS OF BELLY ULCERS

An ulcer is a lesion that develops on your skin or mucus membranes of your body. The symptoms are acute for many people and mild for others.

Key Points

· Notice any pain in your stomach in the middle of your breastbone as well as your belly button.

· Watch for other common symptoms, including: nausea, lethargy, lack of appetite, and weight reduction.

· Watch for more serious symptoms, including: vomiting and dark, tarry, bloody, or pasty stools. You may be vulnerable if you: regularly take nonsteroidal anti-inflammatory drugs, have a family group background of ulcers, have illnesses from the liver organ, kidney, or lung, or are more than 50 years.

Recognizing Symptoms

1 Focus on pain in your belly ranging from your breastbone as well as your belly button. The pain may differ in intensity and duration, enduring from a short while to many hours. It often occurs between foods as your abdomen empties, and could certainly be a burning, aching or stabbing pain.

· Often pain triggered by ulcers can be temporarily relieved by consuming foods that buffer the acidity in the tummy, or by firmly taking an over-the-counter antacid medication.

· If your belly pain is triggered by ulcers, flareups might occur during the night and once you are starving.

2 Watch out for other symptoms of ulcers that sufferers have reported. Many of these symptoms don't happen for everyone, but you may experience a mixture of any of them.

· An upsurge in the quantity of gas and burping.

· A feeling of fullness and a failure to drink a great deal of liquids.

· Being hungry a few hours after eating meals.

· Mild nausea, most common on first waking each day.

· An overall feeling to be tired rather than feeling well.

· Reduction of appetite.

· Weight loss.

Understand the Symptoms of A Severe Ulcer

If remaining untreated, ulcers can cause inner bleeding and other problems, resulting in a medical crisis.

· Vomiting, particularly if bloodstream exists, is definitely an indicator of advanced ulcers.

· Dark, tarry or pasty stool can also be an indicator of severe ulcers.

· Bloody stools.

See your physician if you are experiencing any ulcers symptoms. Ulcers are a significant condition that wants medical treatment. Over-the-counter products may provide short-term relief, however they do not treat the problem.

Know if you will get belly ulcers:

While abdomen ulcers can present for just about any quantity of reasons, people most in danger to build up them include:

· People contaminated by the H. pylori bacterium.

· People who regularly take nonsteroidal anti-inflammatory drugs (NSAIDs) such as ibuprofen, aspirin, or naproxen.

· People with a family group background of ulcers.

· People who regularly consume alcohol.

· People who've illnesses or diseases from the liver organ, kidney, or lung.

· People over the age of 50 years.

Quick Tips for Persons Experiencing Ulcers

1. Schedule an appointment with your physician. Some tummy ulcers will heal independently, some severe belly ulcers will

would have to be diagnosed and treated with an endoscope. An endoscope is a little, lighted pipe that is installed down your esophagus. Only your physician is capable of doing this. For the time being, try a few of these quick fixes before you observe your practitioner.

2. Take an acid-blocking medication. An acid-blocking medication may also be suggested by doctors to find out if symptoms improve. That's because abdomen ulcers can be triggered by an imbalance between your digestive liquids in the tummy and duodenum.

3. Make certain changes in lifestyle. Stop smoking, and taking NSAIDs. Smoking and taking in can both cause imbalances in digestive liquids, while NSAIDs can disrupt the total amount if used high dosages. Discontinue all three when you are looking forward to an analysis from your physician.

4. Don't drink dairy. Drinking milk may provide short-term relief, but it's like taking one step of progress and two steps back again. Dairy will layer the liner of your belly wall structure for some time. But dairy will also stimulate the creation of more gastric acid, which eventually aggravate the ulcers even more.

Receiving Treatment

1. Identify the symptoms of ulcers. Abdominal problems tend to be difficult to diagnose, because the symptoms of anybody problem are similar to several different types of issues, including gastritis, pancreatitis, Crohn's disease, and a number of other problems. It's important to see your physician and reach an authentic diagnosis if you believe you might have an ulcer, and that means you can have the care. Ulcer medical indications include:

· Prolonged or reoccurring abdomen or stomach pain. Often with pain there is certainly pain or bloating feeling in the abdominal.

· Nausea and vomiting

· Reduction of appetite

· Traces of bloodstream in vomit. Dark or tarry-looking stool indicative of bleeding from top of the area of the small intestine.

· Weight reduction, pallor, light-headed, weakness. That is credited to persistent loss of blood.

Your general specialist may advise that you go to a GI (gastrointestinal) specialist, where time you might feel the pursuing tests which may be used to properly diagnose any type of digestive ulcer:

Non-invasive assessments include:

· Ultrasound entire abdomen

· MRI

· Top gastrointestinal (GI) x-ray series. After taking in a chalky material called barium, you should have x-rays taken up to look for indicators of ulcers in your tummy.

· Once the ulcer is detected, the physician may advise endoscopy to learn the precise location and degree of the ulcer. When you are under moderate sedation, the physician will place a thin pipe with a little camera by the end down your throat and into the stomach. The camera allows the physician to see of one's digestive monitor and tack a cells test. That is a straightforward and almost pain-free procedure.

· Blood tests. These will be performed to check on for growths or antibodies to H. pylori, a bacteria associated with gastritis and ulcers commonly.

· Stool checks with culture is performed to verify bleeding as well as the existence of H.pylori

4. Tackle the main of the problem. Ulcers have to be healed by dealing with the root condition of the ulcer specific for you. That's why it's important to obtain a proper analysis and continue with your doctor's suggested treatment. Most treatments involve medication, removing the reason for the ulcer and diet changes.

· Often, H. pylori contamination is at fault, in which particular case the physician will prescribe an antibiotic to help eradicate it. In some full cases, you might be recommended proton-pump inhibitor like omeprazole (Prilosec) or an H2 agonist (Pepcid), which blocks the creation of acidity in your belly and allows your abdomen to heal.

· In acute cases, surgery may be necessary or if problems develop consequently of ulcers that go too long without treatment.

5. Avoid taking aspirin and NSAIDs. Aspirin and non-steroidal anti-inflammatory drugs (NSAIDs) can cause ulcers, and can exacerbate the symptoms. Avoid taking NSAIDS when you have a dynamic ulcer as well as for prolonged periods of that time period thereafter.

· If you will need to consider medication to cope with pain symptoms, ask a health care provider about your alternatives. In some instances, you may be capable to have a NSAID along with an acidity reducer, or pursue option pain treatments.

Try over-the-counter antacids to help lessen your symptoms. Often you will feel indigestion and acid reflux, with burning up and nausea in the top tummy under the ribs. Antacids may be used to provide temporary alleviation of symptoms, but will not eventually cure ulcers. In fact, some antacids may hinder the potency of prescription medications, so speak to your doctor before taking them. Over-the-counter antacids options include:

· Calcium mineral carbonates, found it products like Rolaids and Tums, is probably the most typical OTC antacid. Sodium bicarbonate products such as Alka-Seltzer and Pepto Bismol (Bismuth Subsalicylate) may also be used to soothe the liner of the tummy, and are available widely.

· Magnesium hydroxide is also common suggested, promoted as Phillips' Dairy of Magnesia. A variety of aluminium hydroxide and magnesium hydroxide comes as Maalox, Mylanta and other brands.

· Less common antacids include light weight aluminum hydroxide, sold under the brands AlternaGEL and Amphojel, among others.

CHAPTER - 4

CHANGING YOUR DAILY DIET

Avoid any foods that aggravate your symptoms. Ulcers change from individual to individual, so it is hard to state what foods are best for ulcers and what foods are bad. For some social people, spicy food could cause no problems, but pastries or olives may drive them crazy with pain. Make an effort to eat a comparatively bland diet while your ulcer heals and identify things that make it worse.

· Often, high-sugar foods, processed food items, fried foods, salted meat, alcohol, and espresso make ulcers worse.

· Increase your liquid intake.

· Try keeping a food diary and jot down everything that you take in per day, to enable you to have an archive of why is it bad, if you start to get a flare up of pain.

· Be judicious in what you trim out for a while to heal up in the long run. A little self-discipline now can help your belly heal quickly and enable you to make contact with a less limited lifestyle.

Eat even more fiber: Some estimations show that the common consumer gets about 14 grams of fiber each day. Make an effort to get upwards of 28-35 grams of fiber per day to take care of your digestive system right. A high-fiber diet which has a lot of fruits and vegetables really helps to reduce your likelihood of getting an ulcer, and helps existing ulcers cure. Try getting fiber from the next sources:

· Apples

· Lentils, peas, and beans

· Brussels sprouts, broccoli, and other brassica

· Berries

· Avocados

· Bran flakes

· Flaxseeds

· Whole whole wheat pasta

· Barley and other wholegrains

· Oatmeal

Eat lots of foods which contain flavonoids. Some research shows that foods made up of normally occurring flavonoids can help heal ulcers quicker. Flavonoids take place normally in many fruits & vegetables, making them good that you should consume on two levels. Good resources include:

· Apples

· Celery

· Cranberries

- Blueberries

- Plums

- Spinach

Try licorice main. Teas and supplements comprising licorice main can help heal ulcers and keep them from returning. It is critical to distinguish between sugary licorice candy, which will make abdomen troubles worse and natural licorice main, which is utilized in supplements and teas. Only use the second option as yet another treatment for ulcers.

Avoid spicy foods like chili peppers or spicy seasonings. Scale back or eliminate those foods from your daily diet.

Highly spiced foods do not reason ulcers; some individuals with ulcers do report that their symptom get worse after eating.

Avoid citrus if it bothers you. Acidic fruits beverages, including orange juice, grapefruit, and other citrus juices can make the symptoms of ulcers much worse. For a lot of, it might not be a problem, but it could be extremely unpleasant for others. Limit your citrus-intake, if it appears to trouble your ulcer.

Scale back on espresso and soda pops. Coffee is acidic highly, which can exacerbate the symptoms of ulcers. Carbonated drinks and colas similarly can irritate your tummy coating and make your symptoms worse. Try to slice out your morning hours sit down elsewhere in the short-term, if you are experiencing an ulcer, to attempt to heal up.

Caffeine in and of itself doesn't make ulcers worse, but acidic carbonated drinks, some strong teas, and espresso do. Try switching to more mild herbal teas, if you come with an ulcer. If you want just a little caffeine kick, try adding some guarana to your tea.

CHAPTER - 5

MAKING CHANGES IN LIFESTYLE

Smoking escalates the likelihood of ulcers developing and helps it be more challenging for existing ulcers to heal. Smokers are twice as likely to develop ulcers as nonsmokers, which makes it critical that you stop smoking if you would like to permit your ulcer to heal properly.

Smokeless tobacco and other types of tobacco include the same, and increased even, risk of belly problems. Try your very best to give up tobacco altogether, if you come with an ulcer.

Chat to your physician about tapering methods, including using prescription drugs to help you ease from a nicotine dependence. Over-the-counter areas and nicotine supplements are also available, which can help.

Avoid alcohol in anticipation of your ulcer is entirely restore to health Alcoholic beverages irritate the abdomen lining, and it requires some time for the tummy to completely heal. If you're dealing with an ulcer, or any type of stomach trouble, it is critical to avoid alcoholic beverages as long as you're recovering. A good ale or two can aggravate your ulcer.

Alcoholic beverages in moderation may be alright in the end treatment is finished, nevertheless, you should discuss it with your physician before resuming taking in virtually any capacity.

Rest with your mind somewhat elevated. For some social people, ulcers can get a great deal worse during the night. Laying smooth on your back again can cause certain ulcers to be more unpleasant, and nighttime is the most severe time to maintain pain. Try seated with your mind and shoulders raised somewhat from the mattress, to remain at a willing position. Some individuals are successful sleeping more soundly such as this, when ulcers are bothering them.

Eat smaller sized meals at regular times. Eating a large meal in the middle of the day can make an ulcer worse. Instead, make an effort to time meals at regular times during the day, and also have smaller meals, instead of a few really big ones. This can help your belly to process small amounts of food easier.

Avoid consuming food too near to bedtime, which can cause nighttime pain that could keep you from sleeping more soundly.

Some people find that the symptoms of ulcers are created worse after eating, while some find that eating can soothe the ulcer pain. Test some with your daily diet to see what works for you.

Be careful in what medication you take. If you go directly to the doctor from here on out, you will need to tell them that you've handled ulcers before, and you would like these to consider your background of abdomen troubles when prescribing medication. Even if you have been ulcer free for quite some time, certain medications can irritate your tummy and make it much worse. Always seek advice from your doctor before switching medications or taking something new.

Give it time. The belly can take a long time to completely heal, & most doctors advise that you have a pretty demanding method of your recovery, and allow an interval of at least 2-3 weeks before you take into account yourself "healed." then Even, a go back to a diet plan or lifestyle that led to your ulcers flaring up to begin with can cause your ulcers another, perhaps more powerful this time. It is critical to commit to your wellbeing and present your stomach enough time it requires to heal.

Some people may heal faster than others, but it is important to continue your dieting and changes in lifestyle well beyond whenever your symptoms subside. Don't celebrate having no abdomen pain with a few beverages, or the pain could come back.

CHAPTER - 6

TREAT ULCERS NATURALLY

Eating Foods that may help you Heal

Eat antioxidant-rich foods. Free radicals in your tummy can breakdown your belly coating, making your ulcer worse. Antioxidants are known as free radical scavengers - they destroy the free radicals that might lead to you harm. As a result of this, you should eat foods which contain antioxidants. Included in these are:

· Red wine

· Pomegranate juice

· Grape juice

· Buckwheat

· Barley

· Coffee beans and lentils

· Nut products (walnuts, peanuts, hazelnuts, almonds, etc.)

· Chocolate

· Berries (blueberries, cranberries, blackberries, raspberries, strawberries, etc.)

· Certain spices (including clove, allspice, cinnamon)

- Certain natural herbs (including peppermint, oregano, thyme, sage, rosemary)

- Tomato products (sauces, sun-dried tomatoes)

Search for foods which contain plenty of flavonoids. Flavonoids are located in much vegetation and are thought as organic substances of natural pigments. Flavonoids also battle free radicals, meaning they may be protectors of your abdomen lining, like antioxidants just. Foods abundant with flavonoids include:

- Blueberries

- Strawberries

- Peaches

- Apples

- Oranges

- Celery

- Dark beans

- Dark, green, and oolong teas

- Beer

Drink cabbage juice. Although it is an unusual drink, cabbage juice is quite effective in treating stomach ulcers. Cabbage is normally abundant with bacteria that produce lactic acidity; these bacteria are crucial in fighting and destroying the bacteria that triggers ulcers.

· You ought to drink 50 ml of cabbage juice double each day when your belly is empty.

· Cabbage juice can be produced at home utilizing a juicer, or can be bought from some marketplaces and health stores.

Consume cranberry products. Cranberry may combat H. pylori. Research in addition has shown that cranberry juice is powerful as it pertains to avoiding bad bacteria from fusing to the liner of your tummy.

· You can drink cranberry juice, eat fresh cranberries, or take cranberry supplements (available from pharmacies and vitamin stores).

· Eat white nice potatoes. Research demonstrates powerful wound-healing agents are located in white lovely potatoes. Eating these can help heal your ulcer. You'll find white special potatoes at many marketplaces and prepare them in a number of ways, including baking and steaming.

·Use more honey. Research and custom demonstrate that honey is a robust natural antibiotic. For this good reason, it can benefit battle the H. pylori bacteria that cause ulcers. Try to consume a couple spoonfuls of honey every day to combat your ulcer.

Take licorice supplements. Licorice main has anti-H. pylori properties, so that it can help heal your ulcer. Licorice draw out is available from many marketplaces, pharmacies, and health stores.

· Chat to your physician prior to starting a licorice routine and discuss other medications you might be taking. Licorice supplements used with diuretics, corticosteroids, or other medications that lower the body's potassium levels could reduce potassium to dangerous levels. Take licorice supplements as instructed by your physician.

Eat even more bananas. Research shows that eating bananas can help treat the symptoms of belly ulcers by assisting to protect the liner of the abdomen. Though you won't heal a preexisting ulcer, eating bananas can help treat your symptoms.

·Dried out unripe plantains also may help, but ripe plantains do not appear to truly have a positive effect.

Change from butter to essential oil. When you'll normally put a pat of butter in the frying skillet to make your eggs or vegetables in, you should instead use essential olive oil. These natural oils contain healthy fat that are prepared easier than the heavier body fat found in pet products like butter.

· You can also try cooking food with coconut essential oil, rice bran essential oil, sesame essential oil or safflower oil

Follow a bland diet. A bland diet specializes in easily-digestible, low-fiber foods. They are mild on your tummy and are less inclined to irritate ulcers.You should talk to your physician about if a bland diet is an excellent treatment for your ulcer, and exactly how long to check out it if it's. Foods you can eat on the bland diet include:

· Low-fat milk products (dairy, yogurt, etc.)

· Cooked, canned, or iced vegetables without seasoning

· vegetable and Fruit

· Applesauce

- Hot cereals

- Lean, tender meat such as boiled poultry or baked seafood, without seasonings

- Creamy peanut butter

- Tofu

CHAPTER - 7

STEPS TO MAKE CABBAGE JUICE

If you have problems with belly ulcers, consider adding cabbage juice to your daily diet. Cabbage juice contains gefarnate and L-glutamine, both which protect the mucous-membrane coating of your abdomen. Cabbage juice is also fermented to produce probiotics that further help your digestive health.

Ingredients

3 mugs (675 g) chopped green cabbage

1 3/4 mugs (435 ml) water

Steps-1

Boil water in a little pot for thirty minutes. To be the very best, the water you utilize should be free from chlorine and other additives. Boiling will rid the drinking water of all unwanted elements, nevertheless, you can also run your drinking water through a filtration system or leave it seated out at room temperature every day and night.

· Note you don't should do this if using distilled drinking water. You merely need to purify your drinking water if it originates from your faucet or well.

Put the cut cabbage and water into a blender. Use a big blender therefore the blender is about 2/3 full. In the event that you fill up the blender to the very best, the ingredients might not blend thoroughly enough.

Mix the cabbage and drinking water collectively at low velocity. Stop when water is green-tinted, with apparent chunks of cabbage still going swimming. This will only take a couple of minutes.

Mix the combination on high for 10 mere seconds. Don't allow the blend to mix at broadband for a lot longer than that. There should be a few small bits of cabbage going swimming in the juice. You don't want to make a paste or a puree.

Pour the mix into a 1-quart (1 liter) jar. Make certain there reaches least 1 in (2.5 centimeters) between your surface of the cabbage combination and the rim of the jar. The liquid will probably increase as it sits, so that it needs room.

Tightly seal the jar with plastic material cover. If the jar you utilize has a lid that will also work very well. For a straight tighter seal, stretch plastic cover over the mouth area of the jar and screw the cover onto the jar on the wrap.

Allow the cabbage blend to sit down undisturbed at room temperature. Avoid allowing the temperature to drop much below 68 levels Fahrenheit (20 levels Celsius) or even to go above 78 levels Fahrenheit (25.6 levels Celsius). The perfect temperature is approximately 72 levels Fahrenheit (22. 2 levels Celsius).

Let the cabbage mix sit down for 3 full times or 72 hours. The juice is fermenting, growing ethnicities that will assist your digestive health.

Place a mesh strainer more than a clean, vacant jar. Make use of a strainer with relatively small spaces, if possible, to split up as a lot of the mixture's water from the mixture's solid parts as you possibly can. Make certain the strainer you utilize is also smaller than the mouth area of the jar to avoid any overlap or spillage.

Pour the pulpy liquid through the strainer and in to the second jar. Stress the liquid gradually to avoid accidentally spilling the juice or leading to the strainer to get clogged with pulp.

Cover the jar. Store your cabbage juice inside the refrigerator until prepared to use and serve it chilled.

Repeat this technique whenever your original source gets low, reserving 1/2 glass (125 milliliters) of your original batch. This 1/2 glass (125 milliliters) should be put into your brand-new batch prior to the fermentation process.

Allow your brand-new batch to sit down at room temperature every day and night before straining. With the addition of cultured juice from an earlier batch, you increased enough time it required for your brand-new batch to ferment.

CHAPTER - 8

STAYING AWAY FROM FEW FOODS

Eliminate alcohol from your daily diet. While alcoholic beverages like wines can involve some health benefits, alcoholic beverages can irritate the liner of your tummy. When you yourself have an ulcer triggered by H. pylori, alcoholic beverages only makes the problem worse.

Don't drink dairy for relief. Drinking milk can offer some short-term relief from pain caused by ulcers because it will cost the stomach; however, consuming dairy will also encourage your belly to create more acidity, worsening your symptoms over time.

Avoid spicy foods. Spicy foods might make ulcers more unpleasant if you currently have one, however they won't cause one. It is advisable to avoid all spicy foods (Chile peppers, hot sauces, etc.) if you have a preexisting ulcer or are predisposed to them.

Don't eat fatty foods. Deep fried foods, junk food foods, and other high-fat foods should be avoided. These fats are hard to break down, which can irritate ulcers.

Avoid garlic. Persons who have ulcers should keep away from garlic that intensify existing ulcers and maybe cause new ones.

Controlling Gastric Ulcer Pain

Reduce pressure on your belly:

As your abdomen has already been under great stress, avoid placing extra physical pressure on your tummy. You can wear clothing it doesn't constrict your belly or stomach. And, you can find comfort by consuming smaller, more frequent meals rather than a few large meals. This reduces the quantity of acidity in your abdomen and maintains the pressure off your tummy.

Try never to eat within 2-3 hours prior to going to bed. This could keep food from placing pressure on your belly while you rest.

Check with your doctor:

There lots of natural methods you can test to take care of ulcer pain. Speak to your doctor prior to trying herbal or home cures. Generally, they're all very safe, nevertheless, you should ensure that the herbal products will connect to any medications you're taking.

Since some remedies haven't been examined for use by women that are pregnant, it is important to talk with your physician about with them if you are pregnant or nursing.

Drink aloe vera juice:

Research implies that aloe vera can help heal gastric ulcers. Aloe juice decreases inflammation and acts to neutralize the gastric acid, reducing pain. To utilize it, drink 1/2 glass of organic aloe vera juice. You are able to sip this each day. But, since aloe vera can become a laxative, limit your consuming to a complete of just one 1 one to two 2 mugs each day.

Make certain to buy aloe vera juice which has a high degree of aloe vera juice. Avoid juices which contain a great deal of added sugar or fruit drinks.

Drink an herbal tea:

Ginger and chamomile make great anti-inflammatory teas which can soothe an annoyed abdomen and reduce nausea and vomiting. Fennel helps settle the tummy and reduces the acidity levels. Mustard also functions as an anti-inflammatory so that as an acidity neutralizer. To get ready:

Ginger tea:

Steep packed tea hand bags. Or, break up 1 teaspoon of fresh ginger and steep it in boiled drinking water for five minutes. Drink ginger tea during the day, especially 20 to thirty minutes before foods.

Fennel tea: Crush in regards to a teaspoon of fennel seeds and steep them in a glass of boiled drinking water for 5 minutes. Add honey to flavor and drink 2-3 cups per day about 20 minutes before foods.

Mustard tea: dissolve powdered or good ready mustard in warm water. Or, you may take 1 teaspoon of mustard orally.

Chamomile tea: steep packed tea bags. You can even steep three to four 4 tablespoons (44.4 to 59.1 ml) of chamomile in 1 cup of boiled water for 5 minutes.

Take licorice main:

Licorice main (deglycyrrhizinated licorice main) is often used to take care of peptic ulcers, canker sores, and reflux. Take the licorice main (which will come in chewable tablets) based on the manufacturer's instructions. You will most probably need to take 2-3 tablets every 4-6 hours. The flavor usually takes a while to get accustomed to, but licorice main can heal your belly, control hyperacidity and decrease pain.

You can also take slippery elm as a chewable tablet or drink (three to four 4 ounces). Slippery elm jackets and soothes annoyed tissues. It is also safe to use during pregnancy.

CHAPTER - 9

HOME CURES FOR A BELLY ULCER

Ulcers in belly, also known as gastric or peptic ulcers, are normal pain illnesses in men and women and in children even. About 4 million People in America suffer from abdomen ulcers, while one Atlanta divorce attorneys 10 American people get an ulcer a minimum of once through the life time (American Gastroenterological Association). They may be open up sores or lesion in the liner of your tummy that are mainly brought on by the acids' discomfort in your belly. Other reasons can be physical damage, alcoholic beverages usage and burns or just the utilization of painkillers like no steroidal anti-inflammatory pills, aspirin, ibuprofen or naproxen. Ulcers can be associated with some symptoms like vomiting, indigestion, stomach pain, nausea, bloating and so on, which make you are feeling irritated and unpleasant. Most of individuals catching stomach ulcers can just suffer from some stomach severe and sharp pain; however, many do not have any sign. If the ulcers become too deep, they can perforate or bleed, which is characterized as vomiting bloodstream and blood moving through the stools. In these severe instances, it is strongly recommended you get the physician examined immediately. It really is known that the original treatment for ulcers in belly is recommended antibiotics that can lead to harsh side results, resulting in many visitors to choose for natural home solutions.

Listed below are top home solutions that certainly help you ease the abdomen ulcers securely and effectively:

Cabbage - Carrots

Cabbage is recognized as among the best home cures for ulcers in the tummy thanks to it are lactic acidity that can produce the amino acidity, which can stimulate blood circulation over the belly lining. Therefore, it can benefit strengthen abdomen coating and heal the ulcer later on. Moreover, cabbage keeps a wealthy amount of supplement C that is found to reap the benefits of patients with H. pylori attacks, while carrot juice comprises vitamin U or named an anti-peptic ulcer factor. The combination of cabbage and carrots would be the first most suitable choice to take care of ulcers in the tummy.

Ingredients:

- 1/2 of the cabbage
- 2 carrots

Direction:

- First, slice the cabbage and carrots in to the small items
- Then, place them in a blender in order to extract the juice
- Next, drink 1/2 glass of the juice
- Do it again this treatment 3-4 times daily (before each food and prior to going to bed) for a few weeks.

A factor to consider is that you have fresh juice every time.

Coconut

Coconut pays to for those experiencing ulcers in belly because of its antibacterial properties. These properties can kill the bacteria leading to ulcers and its anti-ulcer qualities. You are able to consume coconut dairy, tender coconut drinking water, or coconut essential oil, some of which will help you treat ulcers in the abdomen effectively.

Process 1: Coconut Dairy or Sensitive Coconut Water

Ingredient:

- 1 glass of coconut dairy or the sensitive coconut water

Direction:

- Drink the coconut dairy or the sensitive coconut water
- You can also consume the kernel of sensitive coconut
- Do it again this treatment 2-3 times daily for a minimum of 1 week

Process 2: Coconut Oil

Ingredient:

- 1 tsp of coconut oil

Direction:

- Consume the coconut oil
- Do it again this remedy double daily (once each day, another during the night) for about 1 week

Bananas

To be able to treat ulcers in the tummy, both unripe and ripe bananas are advantageous due to its antibacterial chemical substances, which inhibit the introduction of ulcer. Plus, bananas protect the machine because of its capability to get rid of acidity of the gastric juices, which really helps to reduce swelling and fortify the belly coating. Therefore, bananas work home cures for ulcers in your abdomen that you should follow at home.

Ingredient:

1 ripe banana

Direction:

- Eat the banana
- Do it again this at least three times daily

You can make banana milkshakes rather than eating ripe bananas.

Honey

Honey contains potent recovery properties that assist much in treating tummy ulcers because its enzyme, called blood sugar oxidase, can produce hydrogen peroxide that kills parasites causing ulcers. Furthermore, honey can soothe and decrease the irritation of your belly lining. Plus, it can help to fortify the abdomen coating, clear the colon and treat and stop tummy ulcers' recurrence. As a total result, using honey as you of effective home cures for ulcers in your abdomen is your very best choice ever.

Ingredient:

- 2 tsp of honey

Direction:

- Consume the honey once daily on a clear stomach each day.

As you begin to remedy your ulcers, you can consume 1 tsp of honey each day

Banana & Honey

This is actually the instruction to help make the combination of banana and honey for treating ulcers:

Ingredients:

- 2-3 bananas
- 1 tsp of honey

Direction:

- First, peel the bananas and then cut them into slim pieces
- Next, place the small slices in sunlight till they become dried out.
- Later on, grind the dried out parts into powder
- After that, blend 2 tsp of dried out banana powder with the honey collectively well
- Consume this mixture
- Do it again this remedy three times daily for about 1 week

Garlic

Garlic that is always available in your kitchen also offers a capacity for treating ulcers in the belly due to its antimicrobial and antibacterial properties that will keep checking the degrees of Helicobacter pylori bacterium (Fred Hutchinson Cancer Research

Middle, Seattle). Therefore, garlic not only can simplicity the swelling but also prevent ulcers in your abdomen.

Ingredient:

- 2-3 garlic cloves
- 1 glass of water

Direction:

- First, crush the garlic cloves
- Then, eat the smashed garlic
- Next, drink water
- Do it again this treatment 1-2 times daily

Cayenne Pepper

It really is surprising that cayenne pepper can be one of home cures for ulcers in the tummy due to its capsaicin substance can inhibit the belly acids' secretion, raise the alkali's creation and stimulate gastric mucosal blood circulation and mucous secretions.

Ingredients:

- 1/8 tsp of cayenne pepper
- 1 glass of water

Direction:

- Add the cayenne pepper in to the water and mix them well
- Then, drink this liquid double daily in the first 2-3 times.

- Afterwards, you steadily increase to 1/4 tsp of cayenne pepper twice per day for the rest of the week.

You are able to consume cayenne pills purchased at medical food stores. You should take 3 tablets daily immediately after foods in a week.

Alternatively, you can include 1 pinch of cayenne pepper to meats, soups and other savory dishes, which will help you, treat ulcers in the abdomen as well.

Licorice Root

Licorice main is proved to work well with avoiding and treating ulcers in tummy since it can help the intestines and belly produce more protective mucus, which forms a covering for the abdomen coating. Therefore, licorice can convenience the ulcer pain and increase it's healing up process.

Ingredients:

- 1-2 tsp of licorice root
- 1 glass of water

Direction:

- Boil water and then add the licorice main into it
- Let it simmer in ten minutes
- Stress and drink the tea
- Do it again this treatment 2-3 times daily in a week

You can even chew and afterwards swallow 2-3 deglycyrrhizinated licorice tablets three times daily in a week. It is simple that you should look for these 380mg tablets in many health food stores.

Licorice Main & White Rice

This is actually the direction to help make the combination of licorice main and white grain for getting gone ulcers in your tummy effectively and safely at home:

Ingredients:

- 1/2 tsp of licorice main powder
- 1 glass of water
- 1 glass of the prepared broken white rice

Direction:

- First, mix the licorice powder with water
- Then, cover and allow it stay over night.
- In another morning, you add the grain in to the infusion
- Soon after, consume it.
- Do it again this treatment once daily in a week

You are able to eat only white rice that will help you relieve ulcers in your stomach as well.

Slippery Elm

Slippery Elm also acts among the do-it-yourself solutions for ulcers in your belly because its internal bark holds mucilage that not only can soothe and relaxed the pain and inflammation but also really helps to remove the extra fat in your intestines.

Ingredients:

- Some internal bark of slippery elm
- 1 glass of tepid to warm water

Direction:

- First, Grind the bark in to the powder
- Then, combine 1 tsp of the powder with the hot water
- Later on, consume the combination three times daily in a week

Fenugreek Honey

Fenugreek contains powerful recovery substances and health advantages. It could be used for effectively dealing with ulcers in the abdomen due to its mucilaginous substance that can protect the liner in the tummy by covering it and facilitate the healing up process. You may use either fenugreek seeds or leaves.

Process 1: Fenugreek Seeds and Honey

Ingredients:

- 1 tsp of fenugreek seeds
- 2 mugs of water
- 1/2 tsp of honey

Direction:

- Boil the seeds in water
- Then, strain the liquid
- Add the honey in to the liquid and mix well
- Consume the blend afterwards
- Do it again this remedy double daily in a week

Process 2: Fenugreek Leaves and Honey

Ingredients:

- 1 glass of fenugreek leaves
- 1 tsp of honey

Direction:

- Boil the fenugreek leaves
- Then, add the honey involved with it
- Eat the mixture
- Do it again this double daily in a week

Fenugreek Seeds & Milk

Ingredients:

- 1 tsp of fenugreek seed powder
- 1 glass of milk

Direction:

- Blend the elements well
- Stress the mixture
- Consume the strained liquid
- Do it again this double daily in a week

Solid wood Apple

Wood apple is one of the useful home cures for ulcers in your belly that you should apply at home. Real wood apple leaves, or called bael, can treat the abdomen ulcers because of their tannins, which can protect the tummy from excessive acid's secretion.

Furthermore, extracted juice of solid wood apple fruits can help reduce irritation and pain due to its mucilage content. Pursuing is the training to utilize real wood apple leaves for dealing with ulcers in the belly.

Ingredients:

- 2-3 timber apple leaves
- 1 glass of water

Direction:

- Soak the leaves in to the drinking water and allow it stay overnight
- In another morning, you stress the mixture
- Consume this on a clear stomach
- Do it again this treatment once daily in a number of weeks.

Green Tea

Green tea extract becomes among the best home cures for ulcers in the abdomen as it keeps flavonoids.

Ingredients:

- 1 small couple of green tea extract leaves or 1-2 green tea extract bags
- 1 glass of water

Direction:

Boil water and put the green tea extract leaves or green tea extract bags involved with it.

Let it stay static in 10-15 minutes

Then, drink the tea

Do it again this treatment 2-3 times daily

Red Clover Tea

Read clover has been used to treatment ulcers in tummy since it contains a substance to normalize the acids in the belly. Plus, it offers soothing impact and boosts the healing up process.

Ingredients:

- Some red clover leaves
- 1 glass of water

Direction:

- Boil water and place the clover involved with it
- Let it simmer in ten minutes
- Drink the liquid before sleeping
- Do it again this treatment once daily for greater results

Apple Cider Vinegar & Cooking Soda

The combination of apple cider vinegar and baking soda acts as another home treatment for ulcers in your stomach due to its alkaline that can keep up with the pH level.

Ingredients:

- 2 big tsp of apple cider vinegar
- 2 mugs of water
- 1 pinch of cooking soda

Direction:

- Combine the substances well
- Then, drink this liquid
- Do it again this treatment 1-2 times daily for greater results

Aloe Vera

Aloe vera juice can soothe and reduce the burning sensation and acidity linked to ulcers in your stomach. You may use aloe vera juice among the do-it-yourself solutions for ulcers in the abdomen.

Ingredients:

- 2 tsp of aloe vera gel
- 1 glass of water

Direction:

- Blend the ingredients jointly well
- Then, consume the juice
- Do it again this 2-3 times daily

Almond & Milk

This is actually the direction to make use of almond dairy for treating ulcers in the tummy that you should follow at home:

Ingredients:

- Some almonds
- 1 glass of milk

Direction:

- Soak the almonds and then peel off them
- Next, grind them in to the paste
- Afterwards, add the paste in to the dairy and mix them well
- Drink the mix immediately
- Do it again this treatment 1-2 times daily

You can only just drink 1-2 cups of goat dairy daily, which will help you soothe your belly as well.

Cucumber

Cucumbers are also effective home cures for ulcers in the abdomen since it contains cooling and cleaning results. Therefore, cucumbers will help you reduce tummy ulcers and their symptoms such as indigestion and acidity.

- You can eat 2-3 natural cucumbers daily
- You can extract cucumbers' juice using their pulp. Then, refrigerate it. Drink the juice on a clear belly each day.

Ginger & Honey

The mixture of ginger and honey is another natural solution to help ease your ulcers' pain and inflammation.

Ingredients:

- 1 tsp of honey
- 1-2 tsp of ginger juice

Direction:

- Combine the elements well
- Then, consume the mixture
- Do it again this 1-2 times daily

Dandelion

Dandelion or Taraxacum officinale is also a great treatment to cure stomach ulcers. This plant is so special since any part of the dandelion herb may oftimes be used as cure. Ideally, its origins can buy the syrup that pays to for treating belly ulcers.

- Also, you can consume dandelion salad
- Alternatively, you can make the greens or create espresso from its root base.
- You should take this plant for 2-4 weeks and then decrease the amount and finally stop this treatment.

Drumstick & Yogurt

Other home cures for ulcers in belly are yogurt and drumstick. You may use the paste created by these two elements in order to deal with your trouble effectively at home. Pursuing is the training to help you create this paste:

Ingredients:

- 10g of drumstick leaves

- Some water
- 1/2 glass of yogurt

Direction:

- Grind the leaves
- Next, mix the drumstick leaves with water
- Then, add the yogurt and blend them well
- Consume this paste once daily to take care of the ulcers in your abdomen.

Castor Essential oil & Milk

Castor essential oil is another good treatment for ulcers in the tummy that you should follow at home.

Ingredients:

- 2-3 drops of castor oil
- 1 glass of milk

Direction:

- First, mix the substances well
- Drink this mixture
- Do it again this once daily

Indian Gooseberry

Another treatment in the best home cures for ulcers in belly is Indian Gooseberry. Using its benefits, Indian gooseberry becomes effective treatment to alleviate the pain and swelling **triggered by ulcers in belly.**

Ingredient:

- 25ml of Indian gooseberry juice

Direction:

- Consume this juice early each day on a clear stomach
- Do it again this treatment once daily to eliminate ulcers

Ash Gourd

Ash gourd, or white gourd, is recognized as a good natural treatment for ulcers in your abdomen. You may make its juice with the goal of easing your trouble by following a recipe below.

Ingredients:

- 20g of ash gourd
- 1 glass of water

Direction:

- Grate the gourd
- Then, press the grated gourd
- Next, add it to water and stir well
- Consume this solution once daily each day on a clear stomach. You ought to have breakfast time for 2-3 hours later on.

Supplement E

Minerals, nutrition, proteins, fibers and vitamin supplements are essential for human's health insurance and particularly, supplement E is effective with ulcers in tummy. It is exposed that invest the supplement E for 4-6 times, you can improve your health body, putting on weight, healthy organs and intestinal and ulcer maintenance.

- You can consume vitamin E essential oil or pills 1-2 times daily for 4-6 times to start to see the positive effects.

Avoiding Alcoholic beverages and Smoking

Whilst you suffer from ulcers in belly, you should miss drinking alcohol, dairy and smoking for the meantime thanks for some following reasons.

It is certainly known the harms of alcohol consumption whether you are fine or sick due to its high acid.

Finally, smoking can worsen the problem as cigarette holds toxic things that can cause more pain and inflammation and make the ulcers bigger in proportions.

Water

Eating 1.5-2 liters of water daily can help the body hydrated and decrease the ulcers pain in abdomen.

On the other hand, you can drink 1 glass of water made up of 1 tsp of barley lawn powder 5-6 times daily that will help you cure your trouble as well.

By way of conclusion, this is a summary of the best do-it-yourself solutions for ulcers in stomach that can effectively help you who suffer from weak digestive tract and particularly unpleasant stomach with ulcers. However, this short book functions as informational goal, not educational or medical purposes; therefore, you should seek advice from the physician for ensuring long-term alleviation previous to using those remedies in the event you can get allergy symptoms or delicate to any ingredient of treatments.

CHAPTER – 10

ULCERATIVE COLITIS

Ulcerative colitis and Crohn's disease are the most frequent types of inflammatory bowel disease. Ulcerative colitis impacts only the intestines and rectum. Crohn's make a difference any area of the digestive tract.

What's ulcerative colitis?

Ulcerative colitis is a disease that triggers inflammation and sores (ulcers) in the liner of the large intestine. It usually influences the lower section (sigmoid digestive tract) and the rectum. Nonetheless it can affect the complete colon. Generally, the greater of the colon that's affected, the worse the symptoms will be. The disease make a difference individuals of any age. But most individuals who have it are diagnosed before the years of 30.

Key points

1. Ulcerative colitis occurs when the liner of your large intestine, rectum, or both becomes inflamed.

2. Although the exact cause of ulcerative colitis is anonymous, your genes, environment, and disease fighting capability all play a role.

3. Ulcerative colitis is a chronic condition. Treatment usually will involve drug remedy or surgery.

Ulcerative colitis is an inflammatory bowel disease (IBD). IBD comprises several diseases that have an effect on the gastrointestinal tract. Ulcerative colitis occurs when the lining of your large intestine (also called the digestive tract), rectum, or both becomes inflamed. This inflammation produces little sores called ulcers on the lining of your intestines. It typically starts in the rectum & spreads rising. It can involve your entire bowel.

The inflammation causes your bowel to go its contents rapidly and empty frequently. As cells on the top of lining of your colon die, ulcers form. The ulcers may cause bleeding and release of mucus and pus.

While this disease impacts folks of all ages, many people are diagnosed between the ages of 15 and 35. After age 50, another small upsurge in diagnosis because of this disease sometimes appears, usually in men.

Who is vulnerable for ulcerative colitis?

A lot of people with ulcerative colitis don't have a family group history of the problem. However, you're much more likely to develop it if a father or mother or sibling also offers the condition.

Ulcerative colitis can form in a person of any race, but it's more common in Caucasians. Some studies also show a possible hyperlink between the use of the drug isotretinoin(Accutane, Amnesteem, Claravis, or Sotret) and ulcerative colitis. Isotretinoin treats cystic acne.

What can cause ulcerative colitis?

Experts aren't sure why it happens. They think it could be induced by the immune system overreacting on track bacteria in the digestive system. Or other varieties of bacteria and viruses could cause it.

What exactly are the symptoms?

The primary symptoms are:

- Abdominal pain or cramps.
- Diarrhea.
- Bleeding from the rectum.

Some individuals also may have a fever, might not exactly feel hungry, and could lose weight. In severe conditions, people may have diarrhea 10 to 20 times a day.

The condition can also cause other problems, such as joint pain, eye problems, or liver disease.

In most people, the symptoms come and go. Some people go for calendar months or years without symptoms (remission). Then they will have a flare-up. About 5 to 10 out of 100 people with ulcerative colitis have symptoms on a regular basis.

The seriousness of symptoms varies among damaged people. Matching to Cedars-Sinai, about 50 percent of individuals diagnosed with ulcerative colitis have mild symptoms. However, symptoms can be severe. Common symptoms of ulcerative colitis include:

- Abdominal pain
- Increased abs sounds
- Bloody stools
- Diarrhea
- Fever
- Rectal pain
- Weight loss
- Malnutrition

Ulcerative colitis could cause additional conditions such as:

- Joint pain
- Joint swelling
- Nausea and lowered appetite
- Skin area problems
- Mouth area sores
- Eyeball inflammation

Issues of ulcerative colitis

Ulcerative colitis increases your risk of colon cancer. The much longer you have the condition, the bigger your risk of this cancer. Because of this increased risk, your doctor will execute a colonoscopy and look for tumor when you receive your diagnosis. Regular screening helps decrease your risk of colon cancer. Repeat screenings every one to three years are advised thereafter. Follow-up screenings can find precancerous cells early on.

Other issues of ulcerative colitis include:

- Thickening of the intestinal wall

- Sepsis, or bloodstream infection

- Severe dehydration

- Toxic megacolon, or a rapidly swelling colon

- Liver organ disease (rare)

- Intestinal bleeding

- Kidney stones

- Infection of your skin layer, bones, and eyes

- Rupture of your colon

- Ankylosing spondylitis, which involves irritation of joints in the middle of your spinal bones

How is ulcerative colitis diagnosed?

Doctors enquire about the symptoms, execute a physical exam, and execute a variety of checks. Tests can help the physician rule out other problems that can cause similar symptoms, such as Crohn's disease, irritable colon syndrome, and diverticulitis.

Tests which may be done include:

- A colonoscopy: In this test, a doctor uses a thin, lighted tool to look at the within of your entire colon. At exactly the same time, the doctor might take an example (biopsy) of the liner of the digestive tract.

- Blood tests, which look for contamination or inflammation.

- Stool sample evaluating to look for blood, an infection, and white bloodstream cells.

How could it be treated?

Ulcerative colitis affects everyone differently. Your physician will help you find treatments that lessen your symptoms and help you avoid new flare-ups.

In case your symptoms are mild, you may only need to use over-the-counter medicines for diarrhea (such as Imodium). Speak to your doctor before you take these medicines.

Many people need prescription medicines, such as aminosalicylates, steroid medicines, or other medicines that reduce the body's immune response. These drugs can stop or reduce symptoms preventing flare-ups.

Some people find that one food makes their symptoms worse. Should this happen to you, it seems sensible never to eat those foods. But be certain to eat a healthy, mixed diet to keep your bodyweight up and also to stay strong.

If you have severe symptoms and drugs don't help, you might need surgery to remove your colon. Removing the colon solutions ulcerative colitis. In addition, it prevents cancer of the colon.

How will ulcerative colitis affect your life?

Individuals who have ulcerative colitis for 8 years or a bit longer also have a greater potential for getting colon cancer. The much longer you experienced ulcerative colitis, the greater your risk. Talk to your doctor about your dependence on cancer screening process. These lab tests help find cancer early, when it's easier to treat.

Ulcerative colitis can be hard to live a life with. Throughout a flare-up, it could seem like you are always operating to the toilet. This is embarrassing. And normally it takes a toll how you are feeling about yourself. Being unsure of when the disease will affect next can be stressful.

If you're having trouble, seek support from family, friends, or a counselor. Or choose a support group. It could be a big help talk to others who are dealing with this disease.

How do I prevent ulcerative colitis?

There is absolutely no solid evidence that indicates what you take in influences ulcerative colitis. You may find that one foods aggravate your symptoms when you yourself have a flare-up. Tactics that might help include:

- Drinking smaller amounts of normal water each day

- Eating smaller sized meals each day

- Limiting your intake of high fiber foodstuffs

- Avoiding fatty foods

- Lowering your intake of milk if you're lactose intolerant

Also, ask your doctor if you should have a multivitamin.

What's the long-term prospect?

The only real cure for ulcerative colitis is removal of the entire colon and rectum. Your physician will usually begin with medical therapy if you don't have a severe problem initially that requires surgery. Some can do well with medical therapy, but many will eventually require surgery.

If you have this condition, your doctor should monitor it, and you'll need to carefully follow your treatment plan during your life.

Ulcerative Colitis: Diet Plan and Guidelines

Although there's no one particular diet for people with ulcerative colitis, there are some general guidelines and recipes that may help keep symptoms at bay.

The Low-Residue Diet

For many individuals with ulcerative colitis, discovering the right diet program is an activity of elimination. You eliminate certain foods that seem to be to aggravate your symptoms and observe how you are feeling. Since there are a few foods that are regarded as common sets off, a diet program that eliminates these food types is best. One particular diet is a low-fiber diet, also called the low-residue diet.

The diet is situated around low-fiber foods that are easy to digest and more likely to slow your bowel movements and limit diarrhea. The diet allows you to eat most of the foods that you'd normally eat, while maintaining your fiber consumption right down to around 10 to 15 grams each day.

The body will still get the necessary amount of proteins and minerals, combined with the fluids and salt that you'll require. Since chronic diarrhea lead to certain nutrient & mineral deficiencies, your doctor might want you to include a multivitamin or another supplementation.

Everything you Can Eat

The following are foods that are recommended on the low-residue diet. Understand that many of these foods can still cause flare-ups, so you may need to make some adjustments or get hold of your doctor and dietitian about alternatives.

- Dairy products: up to 2 cups of milk, cottage cheese, pudding, or yogurt each day

- Grains: refined white breads, pasta, crackers, and dry cereals that contain significantly less than 1/2 a gram of dietary fiber per serving

- Meat and other proteins: soft and tender cooked meat, such as poultry, eggs, pork, and seafood; soft peanut and nut butter

- Fruits: fruit juices without pulp; canned fruits and applesauce, not including pineapple; raw, ripe bananas, melon, cantaloupe, watermelon, plums, peaches, and apricots

- Vegetables: raw lettuce, cucumbers, zucchini, and onion; cooked spinach, pumpkin, seedless yellowish squash, carrots, eggplant, potatoes, and inexperienced and wax beans

- Fat and sauces: butter, margarine, mayonnaise, oils, easy sauces, and dressings (not tomato); whipped cream; easy condiments

Avoid the following foods while on a low-residue diet:

- Deli meats

- Dried out fruits, berries, figs, prunes, and prune juice

- Raw vegetables not mentioned in the list above

- Spicy sauces, dressings, pickles, and relishes with chunks

- Nuts, seeds, and popcorn

- Foods and drinks that contain caffeine containing drinks, cocoa, and alcohol

The American Dietetic Association recommends the next eating practices:

- Eat smaller meals every three or four 4 hours.

- Drink at least 8 cups of drinking water each day to avoid dehydration.

- Eat foods filled with added probiotics and prebiotics to encourage better gut health.

- Limit oils to 8 teaspoons a day.

Creating delicious meals can appear challenging when you yourself have to alter your diet and avoid foods. Luckily, the low-residue diet still allows you to eat most of the foods that you're probably familiar with. Bear in mind, having ulcerative colitis doesn't mean you have to sacrifice your taste buds to boring or bland food. When symptoms handle, many people have the ability to consume previously averted foods with higher fibers again.

****

Printed in Great Britain
by Amazon